METASTATIC BREAST CANCER

a review of contemporary state-
of-the-art of therapeutics

DR. BHRATRI BHUSHAN

MBBS, MD (MEDICINE), DM (MEDICAL ONCOLOGY)
CONSULTANT MEDICAL ONCOLOGIST AND HEMATOLOGIST

Copyright © 2019 by Dr. Bhratri Bhushan

A6, Jindal hospital, Hisar, Haryana, India 125001
www.bhratri@gmail.com

CONTENTS

Title Page   1

Copyright   2

CHAPTER 1: INTRODUCTION   9

CHAPTER 2: PRINCIPLES OF DIAGNOSIS   13

CHAPTER 3: TREATMENT OF LOCAL DISEASE   16
AND LIMITED METASTASIS

CHAPTER 4: HORMONE RECEPTOR POSITIVE,   21
HER2 NEGATIVE MBC

CHAPTER 5: HER2-POSITIVE MBC   38

CHAPTER 6: CHEMOTHERAPY IN MBC   50

Dr. Bhratri Bhushan

"Even the darkest night will end and the sun will rise."

VICTOR HUGO

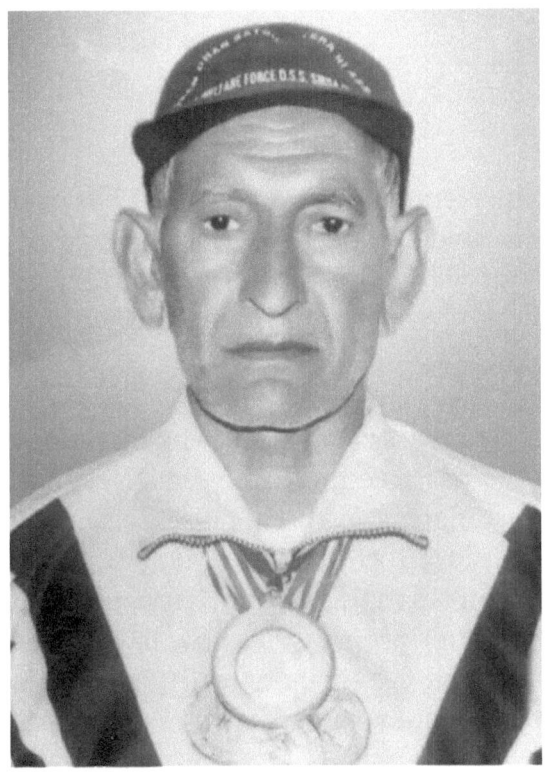

In the loving memory of late Mr. Ram Pal (1944 to 2010).

PREFACE

The tremendous progress that has been made in understanding of the biology of breast cancer has resulted in discovery of many new drugs, giving patients hope and prolonged survival benefits.

Metastatic breast cancer (MBC) is a dreaded disease and in the past the median overall survival of the patients suffering from this disease was 18 to 24 months. It is still the case for many subsets of MBC patients, but in majority of other types of this disease enormous progress has now been made, making prolonged survivals a reality and something which is expected rather than an exception.

The new discoveries include CDK 4/6 inhibitors (palbociclib, ribociclib, abemaciclib), mTOR inhibitors (everolimus), PIK3CA targeting drugs (alpelisib), new HER2-targeting drugs (pertuzumab, T-DM1, neratinib), PARP inhibitors (olaparib, talazoparib), immunotherapy molecules (atezolizumab), new combinations of these and other agents with existing chemotherapy and/or endocrine therapy molecules. Besides these new discoveries, the increased experience with already existing drugs and practices like ovarian suppression/ablation in pre-menopausal women is also translating in clinical benefit.

This book is written mainly for the medical professionals, but it may also serve the general readers to acquaint themselves with the latest developments in medical oncology in the field of MBC management.

I am grateful to my father for his constant encouragement, my mother for her blessings and unconditional love, my wife and my son for giving my life meaning.

CHAPTER 1: INTRODUCTION

B reast cancer is the most frequently diagnosed cancer in females worldwide and is the most frequent cause of cancer related deaths in females globally, although in some nations lung cancer has become the leading cause of cancer related deaths in females as well.

The etiology of breast cancer has been studied in detail and many factors have been identified. Breast cancer is predominantly a disease of females although it affects males as well, so female gender is an obvious associated factor. The vast majority of patients are above 50 years of age, and the incidence as well as the risk increases with increasing age.

Events in lives of females that increase the exposure of breast tissue to sex hormones, predominantly estrogen, increase the risk of development of breast cancer. The events include early menarche, late menopause and older age at first childbirth. Hormone replacement therapy (HRT) has been associated with breast cancer in some studies.

Treatment history as that of receiving therapeutic chest wall irradiation at an early age (like in cases of Hodgkin's lymphoma in the previous era) increase the risk of breast cancer. Bilateral oophorectomy reduces the risk and so does prophylactic bilateral mastectomy, which are most commonly done in patients of hereditary breast ovarian cancer syndromes associated with BRCA1/2 mutations. History of benign proliferative breast diseases and dense breasts on mammograpy impart a higher risk.

Breast cancer once was treated with heroic Halstedian surgeries that spared no extent of surgical resection in order to maximize treatment outcomes. It gradually gave way to conservative surgeries with incorporation of systemic chemotherapy and radiation therapy. Another approach discovered more than a century ago was to remove the ovaries which led to shrinkage of breast tumors, later the biology of this phenomenon was recognized and endocrine therapies were discovered. Then came the HER2-directed therapies which targeted the driver mutation HER2. All this and many other therapeutic endeavours have made this once feared disease very much curable at early stages and even at locally advanced stages.

But there is a subset of breast cancer patients in whom the cancer spreads to other parts of body, thus becoming metastatic. The principles of management of metastatic breast cancer are categorically different than any other stage. Despite all the enormous progress that has been made in the field of management of metastatic breast cancer (MBC), it is **not** considered curative. The intent in such cases is palliative, although in some cases of limited metastasis (oligometastatic disease) cure may be attained in a select few patients, such cases are exceptions and not the rule. Overall, the median overall survival of MBC patients is 18 to 24 months, but it can be much shorter or prolonged depending upon many factors.

MBC is a rare presentation in developed countries with less than 5 percent of total breast cancer patients **presenting** as MBC in the first place, while the reality is very different in developing countries. This infrequent diagnosis of MBC has become possible due to the tremendous efforts put in screening programs that are very effective in detection of breast cancers at early stages. But while the presentation of MBC is rare the progression of early breast cancers to MBC is not so much. In fact, more than a third of early breast cancer patients progress to MBC. Thus there is a huge incidence of MBC patients globally and with the advent and almost universal availability of cutting edge medicine, the patients of MBC are living longer than ever, making the prevalence of this disease higher than ever before as well.

Dr. Bhratri Bhushan

In the subsequent chapters we will discuss the current state-of-the-art of therapeutics of MBC patients as well as pertinent discussion about the challenges faced in resource poor settings.

CHAPTER 2: PRINCIPLES OF DIAGNOSIS

P atients of MBC who present **de novo** should undergo complete history and clinical examination, the importance of which can't be overstated as these may lead to assessment of symptoms and signs elucidated and more judicious and fruitful use of diagnostic tests is made possible. After this basic blood biochemistry, LFT (including alkaline phosphatase levels), chest CT scans and bone scans are to be done. These tests are to be done in **every** patient.

In some patients, depending on the symptoms or a high index of suspicion abdominal (sometimes pelvic too) CT scan or MRI is done. In practice many clinicians resort to PET-CT scan as a one-stop-shop test, but it is in fact not recommended by guidelines. It's not that PET-CT scan is not a good test, it is; and in some cancers like lung and lymphoma it is recommended and is undoubtedly superior but studies in breast cancer patients in this regard are lacking and most of the data are retrospective. PET-

CT should only be used if other studies are equivocal and even then guidelines suggest biopsy of suspicious lesions. PET has limited efficacy in detection of brain metastasis and MRI is more helpful in this situation.

These above mentioned tests are also to be done in patients who were having breast cancer of localized stage previously but are now suspected of being metastatic. In both **de novo** and progressed patients biopsy has to be done. In patients who don't have a history of breast cancer the necessity of biopsy is obvious as we have to ascertain the histological type of malignancy and if it turns out to be breast cancer (breast tissue may give rise to other histologies like lymphoma, sarcoma, phylloides tumor et cetera) then ER, PR and HER2 (more recently PIK3CA, although sampling may be done from peripheral blood is some cases for this mutation analysis) status is to be obtained which is imperative for formulating a treatment plan.

In patients who had a history of breast cancer, biopsy of recurrent/metastatic lesions are needed as well. The reason for doing a repeat biopsy in an established case is the **discordance** found in studies. Discordance means that ER/PR/HER2 patterns may change between previous and current cancer. The rates of such discordance for ER-negative to ER-positive have been reported to be in the range of 3.4 to 60%; for ER-positive to ER-negative 7.2 to 31%

and 0.7 to 11% for HER2. That being said, these tests are not to be followed blindly. Suppose if ER was previously positive but is now negative and the clinical course suggests that disease is behaving more likely as that of an ER-positive one, then ER should be **considered** positive and therapy chosen accordingly rather than the newly found ER-negative status based therapy. Overall, the decision is multidisciplinary and expert opinion may vary.

At present MBC is divided in three broad headings:

1. Hormone receptor positive **and** HER2-negative
2. HER2-positive **regardless** of hormone receptor status
3. Both HER2 and hormone receptor negative (triple negative)

There are many drugs available and approved today, that are being used routinely, that target entirely different mechanisms than the above mentioned three targets. Nevertheless the major deciding factors in selection of therapy are HR and HER2 status.

CHAPTER 3: TREATMENT OF LOCAL DISEASE AND LIMITED METASTASIS

Locoregional recurrence (LRR):
Breast cancer that becomes locoregionally recurrent (LRR) could be treated with a curative intent. Surgery and/or radiation therapy is used for such recurrences and following this, systemic chemotherapy and/or endocrine therapy should be used to minimize recurrences. The patterns of LRR depend upon the treatment plan used in the management of the primary breast cancer. Most of the LRR occur in chest wall and supraclavicular lymph nodes, but other sites may be involved too. The principles of surgery in the treatment of LRR are the same as those of in the treatment of primary cancer, with obtaining margin negative status being the goal.

The role of adjuvant therapy was studied in the CALOR trial. It was a pragmatic, open-label, randomised trial that accrued patients with histologically proven and completely excised ILRR (isolated locoregional recurrence) after unilateral breast cancer who had undergone a mastectomy or lumpectomy with clear surgical margins. Eligible patients were enrolled from hospitals worldwide and were centrally randomised (1:1) to chemotherapy (type selected by the investigator; multidrug for at least four courses recommended) or no chemotherapy, using permuted blocks, and stratified by previous chemotherapy, estrogen-receptor and progesterone-receptor status, and location of ILRR. Patients with oestrogen-receptor-positive ILRR received adjuvant endocrine therapy, radiation therapy was mandated for patients with microscopically involved surgical margins, and anti- *HER2* therapy was optional. The primary endpoint was disease-free survival. All analyses were by intention to treat.

Eighty five patients were randomly assigned to receive chemotherapy and 77 were assigned to no chemotherapy. At a median follow-up of 4·9 years (IQR 3·6–6 ·0), 24 (28%) patients had disease-free survival events in the chemotherapy group compared with 34 (44%) in the no chemotherapy group. 5-year disease-free survival was 69% (95% CI 56–79) with chemotherapy versus 57% (44–67) without chemotherapy (hazard ratio 0·59 [95% CI 0·35–0·99]; p=0·046). Adjuvant chemotherapy was significantly more effective for women with estrogen-receptor-negative ILRR (p interaction=0·046), but analyses of disease-free survival according to the estrogen-receptor status of the primary tumour were not statistically significant (p interaction=0·43). Of the 81 patients who received chemotherapy, 12 (15%) had serious adverse events. The most common adverse events were neutropenia, febrile neutropenia, and intestinal infection.

The conclusion of this study was that adjuvant chemotherapy should be used in patients treated for ILRR and especially so in cases who are hormone receptor negative.

Management of breast primary in MBC:

In most centres around the world, surgery of breast mass is not performed in MBC because data on survival benefit are sparse and whatever data we do have are conflicting. In many trials there was absolutely no benefit of performing surgery on breast on overall survival, while in others there was a benefit that was not statistically significant. In some trials, chemotherapy was first given and patients who responded well to chemotherapy were taken up for surgery and in these patients there were improvements in progression free survival, while in some studies local recurrences were reduced and distant metastasis rates were increased. So the data is not clear and offering surgery of primary site is an exception. Although in some cases doing a palliative mastectomy is necessary as there may be bleeding, a fungating mass or infection et cetera.

Oligometastatic disease:

Making generalized recommendations for such a complex topic of carcinoma breast having "limited" metastasis is not possible. But as a general rule it will be handy to remember that liver metastasis are the most notorious and administering "local" therapy to liver metastasis will most probably not result in increased survival. In metastases affecting other organs therapy directed towards them may increase survival or at least relieve symptoms. But even then single organ limited metastasis only patients are expected to derive these benefits. There is no one-size-fits-all approach in oligometastatic disease management and individualization is a must.

Isolated brain metastasis should be addressed prior to starting systemic chemotherapy as most of the systemic chemo molecules active against breast cancer either don't cross blood brain barrier or do so minimally. Resection is the preferred option if feasible and if not then SRS should be used. Whole brain radiation should be avoided as it results in undue toxicity and SRS is a better available option.

Isolated bone metastasis, especially solitary are amenable to resection if they involve a weight bearing site, and otherwise too. And if resection is not warranted then radiation is a good option. Breast cancer may metastasize to ovaries, and in isolated involvement of these organs surgical removal should be contemplated. This will have the added advantage of removal of a major source of estrogen and will open up the possibility of administering many other therapies if the patient is premenopausal.

Bisphosphonates are used in many settings in metastatic breast cancer. One of the obvious situations is the presentation with single or multiple bone metastasis. Also in patients receiving aromatase inhibitors, periodic bisphophonate administration becomes necessary.

Liver metastasis may be addressed with radiofrequency ablation, directed chemotherapy administration and other methods but the caveat is that the interventions may prove to be morbid and not fruitful in regards to survival outcomes. Lung metastasis may be resected, especially in patients with prolonged disease free intervals after treatment of the primary breast cancer, more so in patients who are hormone receptor positive.

CHAPTER 4: HORMONE RECEPTOR POSITIVE, HER2 NEGATIVE MBC

B reast cancer is not "one" disease. Each patient is unique and the tools for identifying this uniqueness, and thus tailoring the therapy to suit the individual patient, rather than a one-size-fits-all approach, are ever evolving. Presently though, the categorisation of metastatic breast cancer patients is done according to two key parameters: their hormonal receptor and HER2 status.

Its important to note here that if HER2 is positive, then the management guidelines for HER2 positive patients are to be followed; regardless of the hormonal receptor positivity or negativity. In this chapter we will discuss the management of patients who are positive for either estrogen receptor (ER) or progesterone receptor (PR) or both; but negative for HER2.

International guidelines, the foremost of which is

the College of American Pathologists (CAP), have released consensus statements about the interpretation of ER and PR results. These tests are performed by immunohistochemistry (IHC) and if 1% or more tumor cells stain positive then the patients is considered hormone receptor positive. There is some controversy regarding the role of endocrine therapy in patients having 2 to 9 percent positivity but the internationally accepted practice is to start with endocrine therapy in patients having 1 percent or more cells positive for ER and/or PR.

If a patient of MBC is positive for hormonal receptors and is eligible for endocrine therapy, it serves the first principle of oncology very well, which is *primum non nocere* (first no harm). The patients of MBC are considered incurable and cytotoxic chemotherapy has many toxicities that may further compromise the quality of life of the patients, all *without* the hope of cure. Endocrine therapy is great in this regard, as these are mostly available in oral formulations, hence are easy to administer; what's more is that they have a very favorable adverse effect profile compared to cytotoxic chemo molecules.

The therapies targeting hormonal receptors in treatment of breast cancer are collectively called "endocrine therapies" or ET. These can be categorised as: aromatase inhibitors (AI) which are letrozole, anastrazole (non-steroidal) and exemestane (steroidal); selective estrogen receptor modulators (SERM) which are tamoxifen and raloxifen; select-ive estrogen receptor downregulator, the only mol-ecule belonging to which presently is fulvestrant. These are most commonly used in practice but ET in not limited to these alone. Trials have shown that ovarian ablation or suppression has a benefi-cial effect in premenopausal females regarding re-duction in breast cancer risk; in fact, this was the first ever conceived and practised "medical" ther-apy for breast cancer, dating back a century. Testos-terone analogs, medroxyprogesterone, high dose estrogen and many other such approaches that in one way or another manipulate the hormonal sys-tem to control the growth of breast cancer cells, are also ET. But with all these latter therapies, the ran-domised controlled trial data is not strong enough to escalate them to the evidence level which has been ascribed to the former.

The selection between SERM and AI depends upon whether the patient is postmenopausal or not. If AI are given in a patient who has not yet achieved menopause, there will either be suboptimal effects, no effects at all or there may be even be opposite effects on the tumor cell growth. The principle is that AIs inhibit the peripheral conversion of an-drogens into estrogens by blocking a process called aromatization, but if ovaries are still functioning (as is obviously the case with premenopausal fe-males) the mere blockade of peripheral aromatization will not be sufficient for depletion of estrogens in the body; so in these cases either tamoxifen is used or ovaries are suppressed/ablated and then AIs are used.

The definition of menopause has been clearly written in guidelines, the criteria according to the guidelines are:

- Prior bilateral oophorectomy.
- 60 years or older.
- Age less than 60 years; amenorrheic for 12 or more months in the absence of chemotherapy, tamoxifen, toremifene, or ovarian suppression; and follicle-stimulating hormone (FSH) and plasma estradiol in the postmenopausal range.
- If taking tamoxifen or toremifene, and age is under 60 years, then FSH and plasma estradiol level should be in the postmenopausal range.
- It is not possible to assign menopausal status to women who are receiving a leuteinizing hormone-releasing hormone agonist or antagonist. In women premenopausal at the time of adjuvant chemotherapy, amenorrhea is not a reliable indicator of menopausal status.

The "postmenopausal levels" of FSH and estradiol have been variably defined. As a general rule the levels of FSH increase, the physiological explanation being that as ovaries "fail" they produce less amounts of estrogen which triggers the release of FSH from the brain which in turn fails to stimulate ovaries to produce estrogen as they just can't produce it, which increases the FSH levels even more. If the menses have stopped for some time, a persistently high level of FSH (over 40 milli-international units per milliliter, or mIU/mL) indicates that menopause may be permanent. Tracking these results over time is important because these levels can swing widely from day to day. For example, in a normal perimenopausal woman, it's not unusual for her FSH level to be low one day and then quite high the next.

Estradiol is the main form of estrogen found in premenopausal women. A normal level is 30-400 picograms per millileter (pg/mL), but after menopause, it falls below 30 pg/mL. If the patient is taking tamoxifen, estrogen levels can be significantly increased above normal, so the test result may not give an accurate picture.

Novel therapies:

Staggering progress has been made in recent times, in understanding the biology of breast cancer. Some of these discoveries were not conceived primarily to address breast cancer (like that of *cyclins*), but because the biological processes of human body are so intricately interwoven, these discoveries paved the way for new strategies for breast cancer patients. Currently in management of MBC, CDK4/6 (cyclin dependent kinase) inhibitors have a major role to play. Three drugs have been approved in this class: palbociclib, ribociclib and abemaciclib. These are approved in first line setting as well as in later lines. The mTOR inhibitor in conjunction with AI (in some trials tamoxifen too) could also be used in the first line. After having progressed on first line ET, the options include a different ET, CDK4/6 inhibitors (if not used previously), mTOR inhibitor everolimus and, the PIK3A inhibitor alpelisib; all in conjunction with mostly AI, sometimes with tamoxifen too. These newer drugs act on different targets and reduce the chances of progression compared with ET alone.

Rebiopsy:

MBC is usually the result of progression while some cases may arise *de novo*. Hence most of the cases would have received ET in curative adjuvant settings. In cases who progress or relapse after having received ET in such a way, biopsy of the newly developed lesion is necessary as there can be discordance (on an average 15%, vide supra) between the hormonal receptor status of the new site versus old site. Discordances may also be found in the HER2 status, although the rates may be lower compared with hormonal status, nevertheless HER2 ought also to be reassessed.

Although there are many other more prominent mechanisms of resistance to ET, their evaluation is not part of routine clinical practice. Recently, PIK3CA testing by ctDNA on the tumour tissue has come to the fore as a companion diagnostic test to the inhibitor molecule, alpelisib, of the aforementioned kinase. So, as most of the patients would not have undergone this testing primarily, rebiopsy also becomes necessary to obtain tissue for testing for the same. Although in cases where biopsy is not feasible for whatever reasons, it is presumed that the initial hormonal and HER2 status are still valid and in such cases, blood samples may be used for the assessment of PIK3CA, although data are lacking for the latter presumption.

Selection of initial therapy:

Patients with HR+/HER2- MBC are best treated with ET with or without addition of newer molecules, but one must consider the urgency of disease control. MBC can be of many severities, like a patient with a single metastatic deposit in opposite supraclavicular node is an MBC patient and so is the patient with extensive liver and lung metastases. In the latter case like scenarios, it is clinically established practice to start with cytotoxic chemotherapy (single agent or some combination). The rationale behind this recommendation is the goal of achieving prompt cytoreduction and hence control of life threatening symptoms and imminent organ failure. In such patients, after a few cycles of chemotherapy, depending on the clinical situation a switch can be made to endocrine therapy.

If the patient has presented with MBC to begin with, or if the previously received adjuvant endocrine therapy was concluded 12 or more months ago, they are candidates for first line endocrine therapy, preferably in combination with a CDK4/6 inhibitor or some other targeted agent. On the other hand, patients who show signs of progression of the disease while undergoing ET in either adjuvant or metastatic setting or who develop metastasis within 12 months of completion of adjuvant ET should be considered for subsequent line of ET with (preferably) or without a targeted agent. If the patient has progressed on two or more lines of ET, then guidelines are not unequivocal about further course of management and it's dependent upon clinical factors and previous responses.

We have already discussed the utmost importance

of menopausal status in females when deciding which ET to choose. In postmenopausal females, the preferred first line option is letrozole combined with a CDK4/6 inhibitor (palbociclib, ribociclib or abemaciclib). The combination of palbociclib and letrozole was studied in PALOMA2 trial and demonstrated improved PFS (24.8 months) versus letrozole alone (14.5 months); hazard ratio [HR] 0.58, 95% CI 0.46-0.72. Ribociclib and letrozole combination was studied in MONALEESA2 and improved PFS (25.3 months) versus letrozole alone (16.0 months); HR for progression or death 0.56, 95% CI 0.45-0.70 at a median follow-up of 26 months. MONARCH3 studied abemaciclib in combination with letrozole and showed median PFS *not reached* versus 14.7 months with letrozole alone; HR 0.54, 95% CI 0.41-0.72. The response rates with these combinations were significantly higher than letrozole alone. The most frequent adverse effects resulting from CDK 4/6 inhibitors were diarrhea, fatigue and neutropenia. As far as superiority of one CDK4/6 inhibitor over another is concerned, it has not yet been studied and thus it's not known.

The above mentioned combinations are the most commonly accepted and are the best options for usage in the first line. Other options for the first line, commonly used in clinical practice are fulvestrant with or without an AI, fulvestrant with a CDK 4/6 inhibitor or AI/SERM alone. The last option may be used with some confidence in patients with low disease burden and who are medically less likely to tolerate the combination with a CDK 4/6 inhibitor.

Selection of subsequent line of therapy:

When MBC progresses on the first line of ET, further management is not well defined and depends on the clinical context. Options include AI with a CDK 4/6 inhibitor, fulvestrant alone, fulvestrant with a CDK 4/6 inhibitor, fulvestrant with alpelisib, everolimus with AI/fulvestrant/tamoxifen, AI/tamoxifen monotherapy and abemaciclib alone. The principle is that the subsequent therapy should preferably act on a different mechanism than the one used previously, to maximize the chances of obtaining a meaningful response. Another important thing to remember is that if a CDK 4/6 inhibitor was used in the previous plan, the chances are that subsequent or continual use would not be of benefit.

Trial data:

Given the choice between AI and fulvestrant, fulvestrant is considered a better option in both front line and subsequent lines as a standalone therapy; but as some patients may choose an orally ingestible tablet over a monthly intramuscular injection, sometimes AI alone may be given. Efficacy of any one AI is not superior to others and they are considered interchangeable, but without any doubt, AI are better than tamoxifen especially in this regard. The evidence of this comes from a meta-analysis that showed treatment with an AI resulted in an improvement in OS compared with tamoxifen (HR 0.89, 95% CI 0.80-0.99).

Another commonly practiced, but not deeply rooted in data, strategy is to use a chemically different AI upon progression. As we have previously discussed, there are steroidal and non-steroidal AIs; so if one type was used in previous treatment then AI with a different mechanism should be used later. Some analyses show letrozole to be superior to other AIs in general, but long-term data show no particular difference.

In SWOG S0226 trial and the FACT trial, anastrazole in combination with fulvestrant was studied against anastrazole alone. The results of these two trials are different because of many known reasons but the combination is an acceptable option.

In a phase three trial fulvestrant improved PFS over anastrozole (16.6 versus 13.8 months; HR for progression or death 0.80, 95% CI 0.637-0.999). Fulvestrant has a theoretical advantage over tamoxifen because of the unique mechanism of action. It downregulates the estrogen receptor and thus may overcome SERM resistance.

Fulvestrant combinations are also options and considered at par with AI and CDK 4/6 combinations, although in the frontline setting only fulvestrant and ribociclib combination has been approved. The data for fulvestrant in combination with palbociclib, in subsequent line setting, comes from the PALOMA3 trial which showed an improvement in PFS with this combination compared with fulvestrant alone (median 9.5 versus 4.6 months; HR 0.46, 95% CI 0.36-0.59).

In subsequent therapy scenario, MONARCH2 trial showed improvement in PFS with the combination of fulvestrant and abemaciclib compared with fulvestrant alone (16.4 versus 9.3 months; HR 0.55, 95% CI 0.45-0.68).

MONALEESA-3 was a unique study as it explored the use of combination fulvestrant and ribociclib not only in the subsequent lines but also in frontline and showed improved PFS compared with fulvestrant alone (21 versus 13 months, respectively; HR 0.59, 95% CI 0.48-0.73).

With the CDK 4/6 inhibitors, the common theme of adverse effects in the trials mentioned above, was of neutropenia, diarrhea and fatigue.

In a recent randomized, phase 3 trial SOLAR-1, the PIK3CA targeting drug alpelisib (at a dose of 300 mg per day) plus fulvestrant (at a dose of 500 mg every 28 days and once on day 15) was compared with placebo plus fulvestrant in patients with HR-positive, HER2-negative advanced breast cancer who had received endocrine therapy previously. A total of 572 patients underwent randomization, including 341 patients with confirmed tumor-tissue *PIK3CA* mutations. In the cohort of patients with *PIK3CA*-mutated cancer, progression-free survival at a median follow-up of 20 months was 11.0 months (95% confidence interval [CI], 7.5 to 14.5) in the alpelisib–fulvestrant group, as compared with 5.7 months (95% CI, 3.7 to 7.4) in the placebo–fulvestrant group (hazard ratio for progression or death, 0.65; 95% CI, 0.50 to 0.85; $P<0.001$); in the cohort without *PIK3CA*-mutated cancer, the hazard ratio was 0.85 (95% CI, 0.58 to 1.25; posterior probability of hazard ratio <1.00, 79.4%). In the overall population, the most frequent adverse events of grade 3 or 4 were hyperglycemia (36.6% in the alpelisib–fulvestrant group vs. 0.7% in the placebo–fulvestrant group) and rash (9.9% vs. 0.3%). Diarrhea of grade 3 occurred in 6.7% of patients in the alpelisib–fulvestrant group, as compared with 0.3% of those in the placebo–fulvestrant group; no diarrhea of grade 4 was reported. The percentages of patients who discontinued alpelisib and placebo owing to adverse events were 25.0% and 4.2%, respectively.

Everolimus is a targeted agent of mechanistic target of rapamycin (mTOR) which is a part of a bigger signaling pathway (PI3K/AKT/mTOR). Combinations of everolimus with AI/tamoxifen/fulvestrant have been studied and showed good results and are approved, mostly in subsequent lines and some in first line as well. These combinations, like many other aforementioned combinations serve the purpose of circumventing and/or overcoming the resistance to ET.

BOLERO-2 trial showed improvement in PFS with the combination of exemestene and everolimus compared with exemestene alone, in patients who had progressed on anastrazole (7 versus 3 months; HR for mortality 0.45, 95% CI 0.35-0.54), but there was no improvement in overall survival. GINECO conducted another study that showed PFS benefit of combination of tamoxifen and everolimus compared with tamoxifen alone in patients who had progressed on an AI. Recently a phase two trial showed similar results with fulvestrant and everolimus.

When the cancer has progressed despite two lines of endocrine therapy, the decision regarding further management is not elucidated by guidelines and factors like disease burden, performance status of the patient and responses to previous therapies play a bigger role in decision making than available data. Abemaciclib has a unique utility in the scenarios of patients progressing after ET as well as chemo, as it has showed a clinical benefit rate (stable or responding disease) of 42 percent, and median PFS of 6.0 months in the MONARCH1 study, as a single agent.

Lesser used therapies:

Progestins like megestrol acetate (preferably at 160 mg daily) and medroxyprogesterone acetate; estrogens like high-dose estradiol 30 mg daily; androgens like testosterone, fluoxymesterone (preferable to others, at dose of 10 mg BD), and danazol are seldom used and are not much effective. In the era of modern medicine there are many other options available but in resource poor settings clinicians often have to resort to these lesser used therapeutic options

Premenopausal women:

Most of the therapies that we have discussed so far apply to postmenopausal females. As we have discussed in the beginning of this chapter, AI are detrimental if used in a premenopausal women. On the other hand, it has been proven in many trials lately that ovarian suppression/ablation coupled with ET is better than tamoxifen in these patients. Not only does ovarian suppression or ablation makes the usage of AIs possible in premenopausal females, but also makes tamoxifen and fulvestrant more effective. To summarize, if ovarian suppression/ablation is done then the patient becomes practically post-menopausal (vide supra) and thus any of the therapies discussed in the previous section may be used.

Ovaries can be suppressed by use of GnRH analogs or other such drugs and ablation can be achieved by radiation or bilateral oophorectomy. Care must be taken in using methods other than surgical removal as suppression may not be adequate and if the patient is not showing expected response to GnRH analogs then radiation or preferably, surgery is to be done. Checking serum estradiol levels regularly should be routine.

MONALEESA-7 is a unique study involving CDK 4/6 inhibitor, as it not only studied postmenopausal women but pre and perimenopausal as well whereas other trials of CDK 4/6 inhibitors only included postmenopausal females. In this trial 672 pre- or perimenopausal women with hormone receptor-positive, HER2-negative, advanced breast cancer were randomly assigned to frontline ribociclib or placebo to be taken concurrently with goserelin, and either tamoxifen or a nonsteroidal AI. PFS was improved with ribociclib (median PFS, 24 versus 13 months; HR 0.55, 95% CI 0.4-0.69), as was the OS rate at 3.5 years, in subsequent reporting (70 versus 46 percent; HR 0.71, 95% CI 0.54-0.95). This trial resulted in FDA approval of the above mentioned combination in this patient population. In a similar fashion, fulvestrant with palbociclib/abemaciclib can be combined with goserelin based on trial data.

Of course, in patients not willing for ovarian suppression due to whatever reasons, tamoxifen is a viable alternative, albeit not a superior one. On a different note, the quest for newer and more effective therapies in HR+/HER2- MBC are far from over and many new molecules with entirely new mechanisms of action are in the pipeline, making the once bleak future of these patients brimming with hope.

CHAPTER 5: HER2-POSITIVE MBC

MBC is a rare primary diagnosis in developed countries, whereas the incidence is much higher in developing countries. Nevertheless, MBC is a prevalent disease as one third or more of breast cancer patients treated with curative intent ultimately progress to MBC.

One fifth of the patients with breast cancer, as a whole, have HER2 overexpression. In the past this overexpression was associated with dismal prognosis but with the advent of targeted therapies, these patients (even those with MBC) are expected to have prolonged survival. The detailed discussion of HER2 testing and interpretation of results is available on the College of American Pathologists (CAP) website and it's important to keep updated with the recent changes of the same.

It is important to understand that in a patient of MBC who shows HER2 positivity (as per CAP guidelines) any systemic treatment plan ought to include a HER2 targeting drug. To summarize the treatment approach, in an MBC patient who has never received HER2 directed therapy the ideal combination is a taxane combined with trastuzumab and pertuzumab. If the patient has previously taken HER2 directed therapy and more than 6 months have elapsed then again the aforementioned combination is to be used. On the other hand, if less than 6 months have elapsed since last HER2 directed therapy (trastuzumab +/- pertuzumab) then ado-trastuzumab emtansine (T-DM1) is preferred, another option would be lapatinib and capecitabine combination. In the subset of MBC patients who are also hormone receptor positive, there is an option to avoid chemotherapy altogether by using the combination of HER2 directed therapy and endocrine therapy. Now we will discuss these topics in detail.

HER2 directed therapy naive patients:

Patients who either present with *de novo* MBC or progress to it, and have never received HER directed therapy have many options available with excellent outcomes. Previously trastuzumab with chemotherapy was the gold standard and in many parts of the world it's still the better choice, as price of the other recently approved drugs are exorbitant. In some patients with low disease burden and who are not very symptomatic, trastuzumab alone may be considered and in case of progression of disease chemotherapy can then be added.

In the CLEOPATRA trial, MBC patients who had not received previous chemotherapy or anti-HER2 therapy for their metastatic disease were randomly assigned to receive pertuzumab, trastuzumab and docetaxel or the combination of docetaxel and trastuzumab. The median overall survival was 56.5 months (95% confidence interval [CI], 49.3 to not reached) in the group receiving the pertuzumab combination, as compared with 40.8 months (95% CI, 35.8 to 48.3) in the group receiving the placebo combination (hazard ratio favoring the pertuzumab group, 0.68; 95% CI, 0.56 to 0.84; P<0.001), a difference of 15.7 months.

This analysis was not adjusted for crossover to the pertuzumab group and is therefore conservative. Results of sensitivity analyses after adjustment for crossover were consistent. Median progression-free survival as assessed by investigators improved by 6.3 months in the pertuzumab group (hazard ratio, 0.68; 95% CI, 0.58 to 0.80). Pertuzumab extended the median duration of response by 7.7 months, as independently assessed. Most adverse events occurred during the administration of docetaxel in the two groups, with long-term cardiac safety maintained.

This trial established the three drug combination of pertuzumab, trastuzumab and docetaxel as the preferred option for HER2-positive MBC patients. Practical application of this study is problematic in resource poor settings as the prices of such a combination are well beyond the reach of patients and reimbursement also is a big issue. Many times in practice I have to omit pertuzumab. Also, the use of docetaxel results in many dose-limiting toxicities, so other taxanes like weekly paclitaxel are better and equally efficacious alternatives.

The duration of therapy is not well defined. Generally, 6 to 12 months of triple drug combination therapy is given, by this time the best radiological response is achieved, then trastuzumab alone is continued indefinitely (pertuzumab may be continued indefinitely along with it too).

Ado-trastuzumab emtansine (T-DM1) is a unique drug as it's an antibody-drug conjugate. Before a recent phase three trial, it was used in later lines and not in first line HER2-positive MBC. In the MARI-ANNE study, 1,095 patients with centrally assessed, HER2-positive, advanced breast cancer and no prior therapy for advanced disease were randomly assigned 1:1:1 to control (trastuzumab plus taxane), T-DM1 plus placebo, hereafter T-DM1, or T-DM1 plus pertuzumab at standard doses. Primary end point was progression-free survival (PFS), as assessed by independent review.

T-DM1 and T-DM1 plus pertuzumab showed non-inferior PFS compared with trastuzumab plus taxane (median PFS: 13.7 months with trastuzumab plus taxane, 14.1 months with T-DM1, and 15.2 months with T-DM1 plus pertuzumab). Neither experimental arm showed PFS superiority to trastuzumab plus taxane. Response rate was 67.9% in patients who were treated with trastuzumab plus taxane, 59.7% with T-DM1, and 64.2% with T-DM1 plus pertuzumab; median response duration was 12.5 months, 20.7 months, and 21.2 months, respectively. The incidence of grade $\geq$ 3 adverse events was numerically higher in the control arm (54.1%) versus the T-DM1 arm (45.4%) and T-DM1 plus pertuzumab (46.2%). Numerically fewer patients discontinued treatment because of adverse events in the T-DM1 arms, and health-related quality of life was maintained for longer in the T-DM1 arms. This study concluded that T-DM1 showed noninferior, *but not superior*, efficacy and better tolerability than did taxane plus trastuzumab for first-line treatment of HER2-positive, advanced breast cancer.

The discussion done above is certainly readily applicable to patients of HER2-positive and HR-negative MBC; but in patients who are HR-positive there is an option of avoiding chemotherapy and giving HER2-directed therapy with ET. Although data are not very robust but this is acceptable in patients who are having low disease burden, are not symptomatic and/or don't want to take chemotherapy for any reason.

The TAnDEM study explored the use of anastrazole alone versus anastrazole combined with trastuzumab in these patients. Postmenopausal women with HER2/hormone receptor-copositive MBC were randomly assigned to anastrozole (1 mg/d orally) with or without trastuzumab (4 mg/kg intravenous infusion on day 1, then 2 mg/kg every week) until progression. The primary end point was progression-free survival (PFS) in the intent-to-treat population.

Overall, 103 patients received trastuzumab plus anastrozole; 104 received anastrozole alone. Patients in the trastuzumab plus anastrozole arm experienced significant improvements in PFS compared with patients receiving anastrozole alone (hazard ratio = 0.63; 95% CI, 0.47 to 0.84; median PFS, 4.8 v 2.4 months; log-rank P = .0016). In patients with centrally confirmed hormone receptor positivity (n = 150), median PFS was 5.6 and 3.8

months in the trastuzumab plus anastrozole and anastrozole alone arms, respectively (log-rank P = .006). Overall survival in the overall and centrally confirmed hormone receptor-positive populations showed no statistically significant treatment difference; however, 70% of patients in the anastrozole alone arm crossed over to receive trastuzumab after progression on anastrozole alone. Incidence of grade 3 and 4 adverse events was 23% and 5%, respectively, in the trastuzumab plus anastrozole arm, and 15% and 1%, respectively, in the anastrozole alone arm; one patient in the combination arm experienced New York Heart Association class II congestive heart failure.

This study concluded that trastuzumab plus anastrozole improves outcomes for patients with HER2/hormone receptor-copositive MBC compared with anastrozole alone, although adverse events and serious adverse events were more frequent with the combination.

Patients who have previously taken HER2-directed therapy:

The time interval elapsed since the last HER2-directed therapy is the primary deciding factor in selection of therapy in such patients. If more than 6 months have gone by, then patients are treated as if they are HER2-directed therapy naive (vide supra). If less than 6 months have passed then T-DM1 is the preferred option.

These recommendations are based on the EMILIA trial, in which the investigators randomly assigned patients with HER2-positive advanced breast cancer, who had previously been treated with trastuzumab and a taxane, to T-DM1 or lapatinib plus capecitabine. The primary end points were progression-free survival (as assessed by independent review), overall survival, and safety. Secondary end points included progression-free survival (investigator-assessed), the objective response rate, and the time to symptom progression. Two interim analyses of overall survival were conducted.

Among 991 randomly assigned patients, median progression-free survival as assessed by independent review was 9.6 months with T-DM1 versus 6.4 months with lapatinib plus capecitabine (hazard ratio for progression or death from any cause, 0.65; 95% confidence interval [CI], 0.55 to 0.77; P<0.001), and median overall survival at the second interim analysis crossed the stopping boundary for efficacy (30.9 months vs. 25.1 months; hazard ratio for death from any cause, 0.68; 95% CI, 0.55 to 0.85; P<0.001). The objective response rate was higher with T-DM1 (43.6%, vs. 30.8% with lapatinib plus capecitabine; P<0.001); results for all additional secondary end points favored T-DM1.

Rates of adverse events of grade 3 or above were higher with lapatinib plus capecitabine than with T-DM1 (57% vs. 41%). The incidences of thrombocytopenia and increased serum aminotransferase levels were higher with T-DM1, whereas the incidences of diarrhea, nausea, vomiting, and palmar–plantar erythrodysesthesia were higher with lapatinib plus capecitabine.

This study concluded that T-DM1 significantly prolonged progression-free and overall survival with less toxicity than lapatinib plus capecitabine in patients with HER2-positive advanced breast cancer previously treated with trastuzumab and a taxane.

Other options in the patients having less than 6 months duration since their last HER2-directed therapy are lapatinib plus chemotherapy as well as other combinations of lapatinib.

Patients progressing after two or more lines of therapy:

Patients who still progress of second line of HER2-directed therapy have limited options. In these patients first consideration should be given to T-DM1, if not previously used. The basis of this recommendation is the TH3RESA trial. This randomised, open-label, phase 3 trial took place in medical centres in 22 countries across Europe, North America, South America, and Asia-Pacific. Eligible patients (≥18 years, left ventricular ejection fraction ≥50%, Eastern Cooperative Oncology Group performance status 0-2) with progressive HER2-positive advanced breast cancer who had received two or more HER2-directed regimens in the advanced setting, including trastuzumab and lapatinib, and previous taxane therapy in any setting, were randomly assigned (in a 2:1 ratio) to trastuzumab emtansine (3·6 mg/kg intravenously every 21 days) or physician's choice using a permuted block randomisation scheme by an interactive voice and web response system. Patients were stratified according to world region (USA vs western Europe vs other), number of previous regimens (excluding single-agent hormonal therapy) for the treatment of advanced disease (two to three vs more than three), and presence of visceral disease (any vs none). Co-primary endpoints were investigator-assessed progression-free survival (PFS) and overall survival in the intention-to-treat population. We report the final PFS analysis and the first interim overall survival analysis.

From Sept 14, 2011, to Nov 19, 2012, 602 patients were randomly assigned (404 to trastuzumab emtansine and 198 to physician's choice). At data cutoff (Feb 11, 2013), 44 patients assigned to physician's choice had crossed over to trastuzumab emtansine. After a median follow-up of 7·2 months (IQR 5·0-10·1 months) in the trastuzumab emtansine group and 6·5 months (IQR 4·1-9·7) in the physician's choice group, 219 (54%) patients in the trastuzumab emtansine group and 129 (65%) of patients in the physician's choice group had PFS events. PFS was significantly improved with trastuzumab emtansine compared with physician's choice (median 6·2 months [95% CI 5·59-6·87] vs 3·3 months [2·89-4·14]; stratified hazard ratio [HR] 0·528 [0·422-0·661]; p<0·0001). Interim overall survival analysis showed a trend favouring trastuzumab emtansine (stratified HR 0·552 [95% CI 0·369-0·826]; p=0·0034), but the stopping boundary was not crossed. A lower incidence of grade 3 or worse adverse events was reported with trastuzumab emtansine than with physician's choice (130 events [32%] in 403 patients vs 80 events [43%] in 184 patients). Neutropenia (ten [2%] vs 29 [16%]), diarrhoea (three [<1%] vs eight [4%]), and febrile neutropenia (one [<1%] vs seven [4%]) were grade 3 or worse adverse events that were more common in the physician's choice group than in the trastuzumab emtansine group. Thrombocytopenia (19 [5%] vs three [2%]) was the grade 3 or worse adverse event that was more common in the trastuzumab emtansine group. 74 (18%) patients in the trastuzumab emtansine group and 38 (21%) in the physician's choice group reported a serious adverse event.

This study concluded that trastuzumab emtansine should be considered as a new standard for patients with HER2-positive advanced breast cancer who have previously received trastuzumab and lapatinib.

Continuation of trastuzumab with cytotoxic chemo or lapatinib is also an option; so is the combination of lapatinib with capecitabine or other chemotherapy. In patients who are HR-positive the combination of trastuzumab, lapatinib and an AI has been proven in an RCT to be superior and may be considered. But in later lines, it all depends on previous lines of therapy and the responses achieved, thus making generalisations difficult.

The duration of any HER2-directed therapy in MBC is not defined and if the disease is stable, the therapy should ideally be continued indefinitely. It's easier said then done as there are cumulative toxicities, especially cardiac and also the financial burden is enormous. To strike a balance is difficult as guidelines **don't** favor discontinuation of therapy.

CHAPTER 6:
CHEMOTHERAPY IN MBC

Systemic chemotherapy has a major role to play in management of MBC. In patients who are hormone receptor (HR) negative and HER2-negative (TNBC) chemotherapy is the obvious only choice. In patients who are HR-negative but HER2-positive, a HER2 targeting agent combined with chemotherapy is the best approach. In MBC patients showing HR-positive and HER2-negative status, the choice is most of the times ET +/- targeted therapy; but in special circumstances like extensive disease burden, life-threatening symptoms, organ dysfunction and resistance to ET, chemotherapy has an advantage over ET in prompt reduction in tumor burden and alleviating the symptoms associated.

Principles of systemic chemotherapy:

If the patient belongs to any of the above mentioned categories and thus is a candidate for chemotherapy, the ideal sequence of its usage are not defined. Personal experience and centre derived guidelines dictate much of the decision making. General medical oncology principles of selection of chemotherapy depending upon the organ functions, comorbidities, previous lines of therapies and performance status are applicable in the selection of appropriate therapy.

Most centres and clinicians start with single agent chemotherapy and upon progression or occurence of unacceptable toxicity a switch is made to another single agent. In some patients who have good performance status, doublet chemotherapy can be used as it will result in faster control of symptoms by virtue of greater and faster tumor burden reduction. On the other hand, using doublet chemotherapy in patients with low disease burden results in no survival benefit with unnecessary toxicity.

Individual chemo molecules should be thoroughly evaluated for use based upon their merits and potential harms. For instance, it would not be wise to use anthracyclines in patients who have received these drugs previously due to the well-known risk of cumulative cardiac toxicity. In patients with neuropathy taxanes and other such agents won't be a good choice. Platinum compounds may be especially active in patients with BRCA mutations. The list of such clinical vignettes is very long and a subject well covered in standard chemotherapy reference books.

Comparison of chemotherapy molecules:

Taxanes active in MBC are paclitaxel, docetaxel and nab-paclitaxel. All can be used and one is not clearly superior to others and have different toxicities that pose challenges in patients with comorbidities. Docetaxel should be used 3-weekly whenever possible rather than weekly. Paclitaxel should be used weekly rather than 3-weekly. These data are based on survival benefits observed in studies and meta-analyses. Nab-paclitaxel is advantageous in patients having diabetes mellitus, as compared to paclitaxel it doesn't require premedication with steroids. Paclitaxel causes more neuropathy, whereas docetaxel is more myelotoxic.

Anthracyclines active in MBC are doxorubicin, epirubicin and pegylated liposomal doxorubicin. The fact, that these are almost always used in adjuvant setting and the risk of cumulative irreversible cardiotoxicity, is a major hindrance in their use in MBC. These can certainly be used in patients who have not received them before and in patients who have received these drugs previously, it would be better to avoid their usage. If these must be used then a cardioprotective agent like dexrazoxane should be used, particularly if cumulative dose of doxorubicin is more than 300 mg/m2.

Antimetabolites, particularly capecitabine is a very good choice in certain patients for many good reasons; like it results in very low incidences and severities of alopecia, neuropathy and myelosuppression as compared with other drugs like taxanes and anthracyclines. The ease of administration is enormous as it's an oral drug. The property of crossing the blood brain barrier offers a unique role in the management of MBC patients having brain metastasis. Gemcitabine is also a good drug as the side effect profile is favorable.

Many other drugs like vinca alkaloids, eribulin, platinum compounds et cetera could also be used; although their use is not routine.

Combinations:

As we have discussed combination chemotherapy protocols (most of the time doublets) offer greater response rates with increased toxicities. Some studies have shown a progression free survival benefit but overall survival benefit either is not there or is not significant. So the treating oncologist must balance between the urgency to obtain a response and the toxicities that will be inherent, in the face of no apparent survival advantage with the

Dr. Bhratri Bhushan

use of concurrent rather than sequential administration of chemotherapy molecules.

The combinations are just too many and standard
guidelines provide such protocols. It all depends on
the clinical context and no protocol has proven superiority over another. The principles of choosing a
single agent are also applicable in this regard. Platinum compound based combinations are thought
to be more effective in HR-negative/HER2-negative
(triple negative) MBC, although this may not be re-
flective of a sound RCT based data but the evidence
in this direction is definitely there.

BRCA associated breast cancers:

Around five percent of patients of breast cancer
have germline BRCA mutation. BRCA1 mutation
leads to triple negative breast cancers and BRCA2
results in tumors expressing ER, but there may be
exceptions. Many times these patients have a fam-
ily history of breast cancer and present at a younger
age.

As most of the cases are triple negative, targeted
therapy is currently not available for the same
and in these patients PARP-inhibitors have shown
benefit. OlympiAD trial studied the use of PARP inhibitor olaparib in this setting. In this phase three

trial olaparib monotherapy was compared with standard therapy in patients with a germline *BRCA* mutation and human epidermal growth factor receptor type 2 (HER2)–negative metastatic breast cancer who had received no more than two previous chemotherapy regimens for metastatic disease. Patients were randomly assigned, in a 2:1 ratio, to receive olaparib tablets (300 mg twice daily) or standard therapy with single-agent chemotherapy of the physician's choice (capecitabine, eribulin, or vinorelbine in 21-day cycles). The primary endpoint was progression-free survival, which was assessed by blinded independent central review and was analyzed on an intention-to-treat basis. Of the 302 patients who underwent randomization, 205 were assigned to receive olaparib and 97 were assigned to receive standard therapy. Median progression-free survival was significantly longer in the olaparib group than in the standard-therapy group (7.0 months vs. 4.2 months; hazard ratio for disease progression or death, 0.58; 95% confidence interval, 0.43 to 0.80; P<0.001). The response rate was 59.9% in the olaparib group and 28.8% in the standard-therapy group. The rate of grade 3 or higher adverse events was 36.6% in the olaparib group and 50.5% in the standard-therapy group, and the rate of treatment discontinuation due to toxic effects was 4.9% and 7.7%, respectively.

This trial concluded that among patients with

HER2-negative metastatic breast cancer and a germline *BRCA* mutation, olaparib monotherapy provided a significant benefit over standard therapy; median progression-free survival was 2.8 months longer and the risk of disease progression or death was 42% lower with olaparib monotherapy than with standard therapy.

Another trial studied a different PARP inhibitor, talazoparib (EMBRACA trial) in a similar fashion as OlympiAD trial and found almost similar results. Median progression-free survival was significantly longer in the talazoparib group than in the standard-therapy group (8.6 months vs. 5.6 months; hazard ratio for disease progression or death, 0.54; 95% confidence interval [CI], 0.41 to 0.71; P<0.001). The interim median hazard ratio for death was 0.76 (95% CI, 0.55 to 1.06; P=0.11 [57% of projected events]). The objective response rate was higher in the talazoparib group than in the standard-therapy group (62.6% vs. 27.2%; odds ratio, 5.0; 95% CI, 2.9 to 8.8; P<0.001).

Role of immunotherapy:

In patients with triple negative metastatic breast cancer (TNBC) the systemic therapy options are very limited. In contrast with HR-positive or HER2-positive patients, who have many targeted drugs available and approved, oncologists have to resort to conventional cytotoxic chemo in TNBC patients. The limited options reflect the dismal survival figures in these patients with average overall survival being less than 18 months.

Immunotherapy has resulted in paradigm shift in management of many cancers, like lung and melanoma but data in breast cancer are not robust. A recently done trial, IMpassion 130, has shown hope in the application of immunotherapy in breast cancer patients. In this phase 3 trial, they randomly assigned (in a 1:1 ratio) patients with untreated metastatic triple-negative breast cancer to receive atezolizumab plus nab-paclitaxel or placebo plus nab-paclitaxel; patients continued the intervention until disease progression or an unacceptable level of toxic effects occurred. Stratification factors were the receipt or nonreceipt of neoadjuvant or adjuvant taxane therapy, the presence or absence of liver metastases at baseline, and programmed death ligand 1 (PD-L1) expression at baseline (positive vs. negative). The two primary endpoints were progression-free survival (in the intention-to-treat population and PD-L1–positive subgroup) and overall survival (tested in the intention-to-treat population; if the finding was significant, then it would be tested in the PD-L1–positive subgroup).

Each group included 451 patients (median follow-up, 12.9 months). In the intention-to-treat analysis, the median progression-free survival was 7.2 months with atezolizumab plus nab-paclitaxel, as compared with 5.5 months with placebo plus nab-paclitaxel (hazard ratio for progression or death, 0.80; 95% confidence interval [CI], 0.69 to 0.92; P=0.002); among patients with PD-L1–positive tumors, the median progression-free survival was 7.5 months and 5.0 months, respectively (hazard ratio, 0.62; 95% CI, 0.49 to 0.78; P<0.001). In the intention-to-treat analysis, the median overall survival was 21.3 months with atezolizumab plus nab-paclitaxel and 17.6 months with placebo plus nab-paclitaxel (hazard ratio for death, 0.84; 95% CI, 0.69 to 1.02; P=0.08); among patients with PD-L1–positive tumors, the median overall survival was 25.0 months and 15.5 months, respectively (hazard ratio, 0.62; 95% CI, 0.45 to 0.86). No new adverse effects were identified. Adverse events that led to the discontinuation of any agent occurred in 15.9% of the patients who received atezolizumab plus nab-paclitaxel and in 8.2% of those who received placebo plus nab-paclitaxel.

This trial concluded that atezolizumab plus nab-paclitaxel prolonged progression-free survival among patients with metastatic triple-negative breast cancer in both the intention-to-treat population and the PD-L1–positive subgroup.

Duration of treatment:

There is no fixed duration of treatment applicable to all patients. The first principle of oncology (*primum non nocere*) plays a bigger part in deciding the treatment duration rather than the anticipated effects of chemotherapy on tumor tissue. If the toxicities are impairing the quality of life of the patient then it will not be prudent to continue giving such therapy and palliative care alone may be continued. On the other hand, if the patient is having a good performance status, the toxicities are not prohibitive and there is willingness on the part of the patient for enduring the mild to moderate adverse effects of chemotherapy, in the face of improbable improvements in overall survival, then chemotherapy may be continued indefinitely. If such an approach is chosen then reassessment should be done every 2 cycles of chemotherapy and oncologist should proceed accordingly.